BREAST CANCER DIET COOKBOOK FOR SENIORS

Healthy Recipes for Recovery, Prevention, and
Wellness.
(With Colorful Pictures)

Dr. Esther Emmanuel

TABLE OF CONTENTS

INTRODUCTION **5**

CHAPTER 1: IMPORTANCE OF NUTRITION DURING CANCER TREATMENT 8

Goals and scope of the cookbook 9

Overview of the breast cancer diet 11

Key nutrients for breast cancer patients 12

Foods to Avoid 14

Meal Planning Tips 17

CHAPTER 2: BREAKFAST RECIPES 20

Berry Smoothie Bowl 20

Avocado Toast with Egg 21

Oatmeal with Berries 23

Greek Yogurt Parfait 25

Quinoa Breakfast Bowl 26

Veggie Omelet 27

Chia Seed Pudding 29

Breakfast Salad 30

Sweet Potato Hash 31

Tofu Scramble 33

CHAPTER 3: LUNCH RECIPES 36

Grilled Chicken Salad 36

Vegetable Soup 38

Quinoa and Kale Salad 39

Tuna and Avocado Salad 41

Greek Yogurt and Berry Parfait 42

Lentil Soup 43

Salmon and Sweet Potato Patties 45
Turkey and Veggie Wrap... 46
CHAPTER 4: DINNER RECIPES.. 48
Baked Salmon 48
Roasted Vegetables and Chicken 49
Zucchini Noodles with Tomato Sauce................................... 50
Grilled Chicken and Asparagus.. 52
Spaghetti Squash with Turkey Bolognese 54
Quinoa Stuffed Bell Peppers.. 56
Eggplant Parmesan 59
Lentil and Vegetable Stir Fry... 60
Turkey Chili 62
CHAPTER 5: SNACK AND DESSERT RECIPES 65
Baked Cinnamon Apple Chips.. 65
Chocolate Avocado Pudding.. 66
Quinoa and Vegetable Salad.. 67
Blueberry Oat Bars... 69
Sweet Potato Brownies 71
CHAPTER 6: 21 DAYS MEAL PLAN 73
Grocery shopping and meal prep tips 80
CONCLUSION... **83**
Additional resources and cookbooks 83

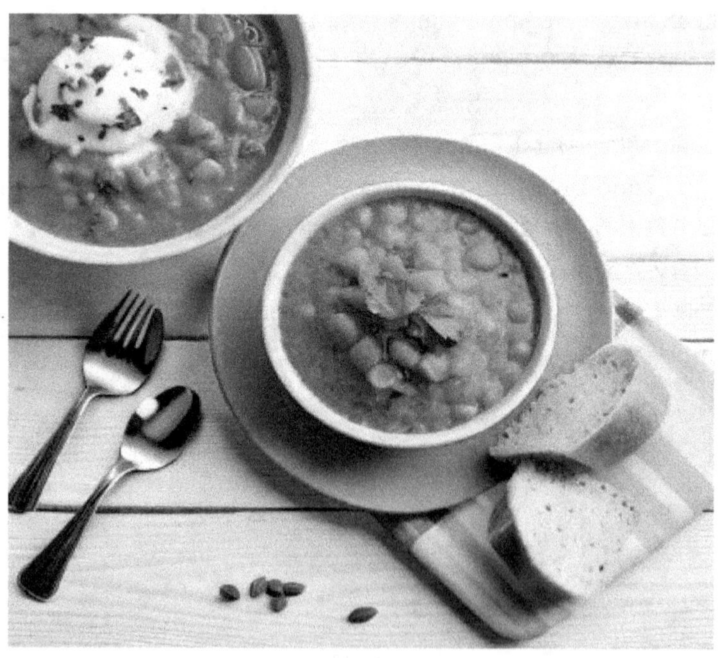

INTRODUCTION

Mrs. Thompson, a woman in her 80s, had been told she had breast cancer. She had always been concerned about her health, controlling what she ate and working out frequently. She was therefore taken aback when her doctor informed her that she had cancer.

Mrs. Thompson, who had always been a fighter, made the decision to attack this obstacle head-on. She started her chemotherapy and radiation treatments right away, but they made her feel exhausted and weak. She began to lose her appetite and was more and more reliant on medicines.

One day, a friend advised Mrs. Thompson that she might consider treating her disease holistically. She was first dubious, but she made the decision to give it a shot. She got in touch with a dietician known for using nutritional therapy to treat cancer patients.

She received a diet recommendation from the nutritionist that comprised whole meals, fresh fruits, and vegetables. Mrs. Thompson was taken aback by how much she could eat on this diet at first, but she soon discovered that the food was not only filling but also tasty.

After only one week on her new diet, Mrs. Thompson noticed a noticeable improvement in her general health.

She had more energy, and her nighttime sleep had improved. She also found that she needed less medicines because her pain levels had subsided.

Mrs. Thompson noticed something even more astonishing as she kept up her diet: her cancer was becoming smaller! Regular checks with the doctor revealed that the tumor was shrinking over time. Her doctor was astounded and enquired as to what she had changed.

Mrs. Thompson explained to her doctor how she had adopted a holistic approach and how her diet had altered to incorporate more fresh vegetables and complete foods. Her physician expressed admiration and concurred that the nutrition therapy was assisting her body in battling the malignancy.

Mrs. Thompson's cancer gradually disappeared until it was completely gone. The outcomes astounded her doctor, who referred to her case as a "miracle." Mrs. Thompson was appreciative of the food therapy that had aided her recovery and she kept up the diet even after the cancer had disappeared.

The Story of Mrs. Thompson was very astounding and demonstrated how often the most straightforward fixes are the best. She was a living example of how altering one's food and lifestyle could result in a recovery from a potentially fatal illness.

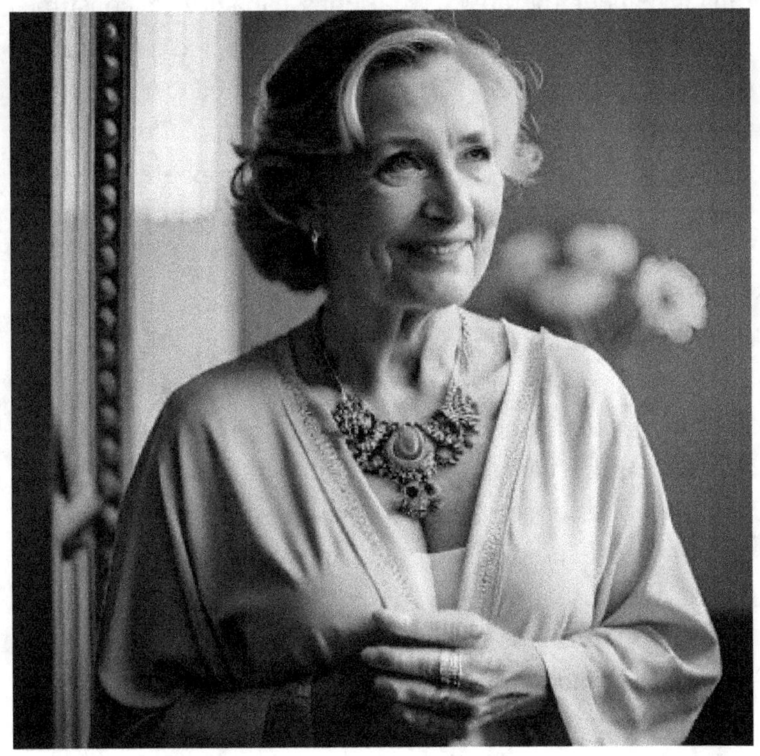

CHAPTER 1

IMPORTANCE OF NUTRITION DURING CANCER TREATMENT

It is impossible to overestimate the significance of diet during cancer therapy. A patient's capacity to consume, digest, and absorb nutrition may be impacted by a variety of adverse effects associated with cancer and its treatments. These adverse effects may include diarrhea, constipation, mouth sores, altered taste, appetite decrease, and weight loss.

For a number of reasons, it's crucial to maintain a healthy diet while receiving cancer treatment. First off, a healthy diet can assist the immune system, which is essential for battling cancer and avoiding infections. Furthermore, healthy eating can support patients in maintaining their strength and energy levels, which can enhance their capacity to handle the mental and physical demands of cancer therapy.

Additionally, a patient's general quality of life can be enhanced and treatment-related adverse effects can be reduced with a good diet. As an illustration, consuming foods high in fiber can aid in preventing constipation, while staying away from acidic and spicy foods can aid in preventing mouth sores and heartburn. Dehydration can be a common adverse effect of chemotherapy and radiation treatment; drinking adequate water can help prevent it.

A balanced diet that includes lots of fruits, vegetables, whole grains, lean proteins, and healthy fats is what cancer patients should try to eat. Eating several modest meals throughout the day as opposed to a few large ones may also be beneficial. To satisfy their unique demands, patients may occasionally need to adjust their diets or use specialist nutritional supplements.

Overall, a patient's ability to retain their health, vitality, and general well-being during this trying period can be aided by excellent nutrition, which is an essential component of cancer treatment. A specialized nutrition plan that takes into account the patient's particular requirements and preferences should be created in collaboration with a healthcare professional or registered dietitian.

Goals and scope of the cookbook

The goal and scope of a senior breast cancer diet cookbook would be to offer a thorough resource for seniors who are receiving breast cancer treatment and are looking for advice on how to maintain a healthy diet during their treatment course.

The cookbook would strive to offer useful, simple recipes that are catered to the unique dietary requirements of elderly people with breast cancer. The meals would be created with the nutrients that seniors with breast cancer require to boost their immune systems, maintain their health and energy levels, and lessen treatment-related adverse effects in mind. They would also be tasty, fulfilling, and simple to prepare.

The cookbook's content would cover breakfast, lunch, supper, snacks, and dessert recipes as well as advice and resources for staying healthy while receiving cancer treatment. The recipes would be based on a breast cancer diet that prioritizes whole, nutrient-dense foods rich in antioxidants, fiber, and other nutrients that fight cancer while minimizing foods that are high in sugar, saturated fat, and processed ingredients.

The major goal and scope of a breast cancer diet cookbook for seniors would be to offer a useful tool that can assist seniors with breast cancer in maintaining a healthy diet and enhancing their general quality of life while undergoing treatment. The cookbook can be a crucial weapon in the fight against breast cancer by providing helpful tips and simple-to-follow recipes that are customized to the special requirements of seniors with breast cancer

Overview of the breast cancer diet

The goal of the breast cancer diet is to encourage optimal nutrition both during and after breast cancer therapy. The breast cancer diet aims to assist breast cancer patients in maintaining their strength, managing treatment side effects, and enhancing their general health and wellbeing.

A balanced, nutrient-rich diet with lots of fruits, vegetables, whole grains, lean proteins, and healthy fats is the foundation of the breast cancer diet. It's critical to select foods that are rich in fiber, antioxidants, and other cancer-preventing components. Several instances of these nutrients are as follows:

- Antioxidants are chemical substances that are present in a variety of fruits and vegetables and can help shield cells from harm brought on by free radicals, unstable molecules that can promote the growth of cancer. Fruits and vegetables with high levels of antioxidants include berries, leafy greens, citrus fruits, and nuts.

- Fiber: This fiber helps keep the digestive system healthy and lowers the chance of developing some cancers. Whole grains, beans, lentils, fruits, and vegetables are examples of foods high in fiber.

- Omega-3 fatty acids: These beneficial fats may lessen bodily inflammation and offer breast cancer protection. Fatty fish (such as salmon and tuna), flaxseed, chia seeds, and walnuts are all excellent sources of omega-3s.

The breast cancer diet also places a strong emphasis on the need to limit or stay away from particular food groups, such as those that are heavy in sugar, saturated fat, and processed items. This is due to the fact that these meals may contribute to bodily inflammation, which may raise the chance of developing cancer.

Overall, the breast cancer diet is made to give patients the nutrients they require to boost their immune systems, keep up their strength and energy levels, and control adverse effects from treatment. Patients can contribute to improve their health and wellbeing both during and after breast cancer treatment by selecting nutrient-dense foods and avoiding those that may be harmful.

Key nutrients for breast cancer patients

In order to promote their health both before and after treatment, breast cancer patients have certain nutritional requirements that must be met. Patients with breast cancer should pay particular attention to the following nutrients:

1. Protein: Protein is necessary for the body to create and repair tissues, and it is especially crucial for breast cancer patients who may endure muscle loss and weakness as a result of their therapy. Lean meats, fish, eggs, dairy products, beans, nuts, and seeds are all excellent sources of protein.

2. Foods high in fiber can lower the chance of developing certain cancers, including breast cancer. Additionally, fiber encourages healthy digestion, which might be crucial for individuals who are experiencing constipation or other digestive problems while receiving therapy. Fruits, vegetables, whole grains, beans, and lentils are excellent sources of fiber.

3. Antioxidants: Antioxidants are crucial for shielding cells from free radical damage, which can hasten the onset of cancer. Berries, leafy greens, citrus fruits, nuts, and seeds are among foods that are high in antioxidants.

4. Omega-3 fatty acids: These beneficial fats have the potential to lower inflammation in the body and may even be protective against breast cancer. Fatty fish (such as salmon and tuna), flaxseed, chia seeds, and walnuts are all excellent sources of omega-3s.

5. Calcium and vitamin D are crucial for supporting bone health, which is susceptible to damage during breast cancer treatment. Dairy products, leafy greens, and fortified foods like tofu and orange juice are all excellent sources of calcium. Sunlight exposure and dietary sources including fatty fish, egg yolks, and fortified meals are two ways to get vitamin D.

It's crucial for breast cancer patients to collaborate with a medical professional or certified dietitian to create a custom nutrition plan that suits their individual requirements and preferences. Additionally, they can assist in making sure that patients get enough of these essential nutrients to support their health and wellbeing both during and after treatment.

Foods to Avoid

While many foods can be helpful for breast cancer patients, some should be avoided or consumed in moderation while undergoing treatment. Here are a few instances:

1. Alcohol: Drinking alcohol has been associated with a higher risk of developing breast cancer and may reduce the efficiency of some cancer

therapies. Alcohol use should be restricted or avoided entirely when receiving treatment for breast cancer.

2. Red meat and processed meat: Deli meats, hot dogs, and bacon are examples of processed meats that are high in preservatives and sodium and have been associated with an increased risk of cancer. Due to the significant amount of saturated fat in red meat, which can fuel the body's inflammatory processes, it should also be consumed in moderation. Lean protein foods including poultry, fish, beans, and nuts are ideal for breast cancer patients.

3. Foods heavy in sugar and saturated fat can cause weight gain and inflammation in the body, which can raise the risk of a cancer recurrence. Patients with breast cancer should avoid processed snacks, sweets, and high-fat diets such as fried foods and fatty meat cuts.

4. Products made from soy: Although soy meals like tofu and soy milk are generally regarded as healthy, there has been some worry that they can interact with some cancer treatments. Before using soy products, breast cancer patients should see

their doctor. They may need to restrict their intake or stop using them completely.

5. Foods that are raw or undercooked should be avoided by breast cancer patients as they may be more susceptible to infection as a result of their treatment. Examples include raw fish, raw eggs, and undercooked meat. These foods might have dangerous bacteria in them that make people sick.

6. Caffeine: Some breast cancer patients may be counseled to consume less caffeine since it may interact with some cancer treatments and aggravate anxiety or sleep problems. Before ingesting caffeinated foods or beverages, breast cancer patients should consult their healthcare professional.

Before making significant dietary changes, breast cancer patients should always speak with their doctor or a trained dietitian because dietary limitations might vary based on the patient and their treatment plan.

Meal Planning Tips

As it can assist ensure that they are obtaining the nutrients they need to sustain their health during treatment, meal planning can be a crucial tool for breast cancer patients.

For people with breast cancer, the following advice on meal preparation:

1. Plan ahead: Making meals in advance can help patients have wholesome options available when they need them and save time. To keep organized, patients might make a weekly menu plan and shopping list.

2. Focus on nutrient-dense foods: People with breast cancer should make an effort to eat a variety of nutrient-dense foods every day, such as whole grains, fruits, vegetables, lean protein sources, and healthy fats. The nutrients that are required to promote general health and wellbeing while undergoing treatment can be found in these foods.

3. Prepare meals in advance: Patients who are suffering fatigue or other side effects of treatment may find it beneficial to prepare meals in advance. Patients can either prepare components in advance to make meal preparation simpler or prepare meals in bulk and freeze them for later use.

4. Utilize leftovers: Making sandwiches, salads, or soups with leftovers is a quick and simple method to produce healthful meals. Patients can also

assemble fresh meals from leftovers, for example, using leftover chicken to make a stir-fry or salad.

5. Use your imagination when it comes to seasoning; breast cancer patients may suffer changes in taste and appetite while undergoing treatment, so utilizing herbs, spices, and other seasonings can help make meals more enjoyable. Patients can experiment with various tastes and textures to discover new foods they like.

6. Remain hydrated: Remaining hydrated is crucial for general health and wellbeing, particularly when receiving treatment for cancer. To assist avoid dehydration and other treatment-related adverse effects, patients should try to drink lots of water and other hydrating liquids throughout the day.

7. Think about collaborating with a certified dietitian: A registered dietitian can assist breast cancer patients in developing a customized meal plan that suits their unique requirements and preferences. Additionally, they can offer advice on how to manage side effects of therapy and maximize nutrient intake.

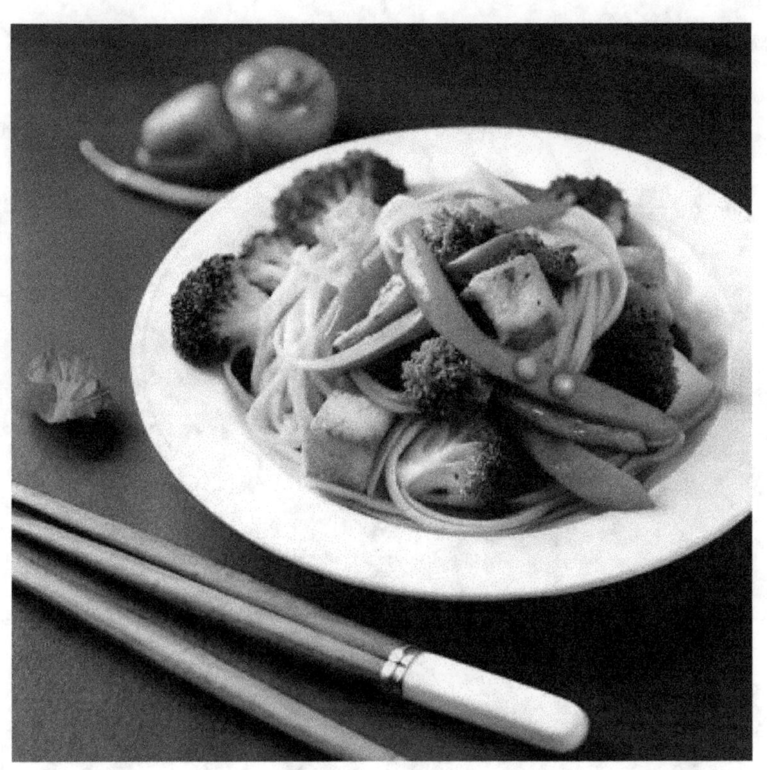

CHAPTER 2

BREAKFAST RECIPES

Berry Smoothie Bowl

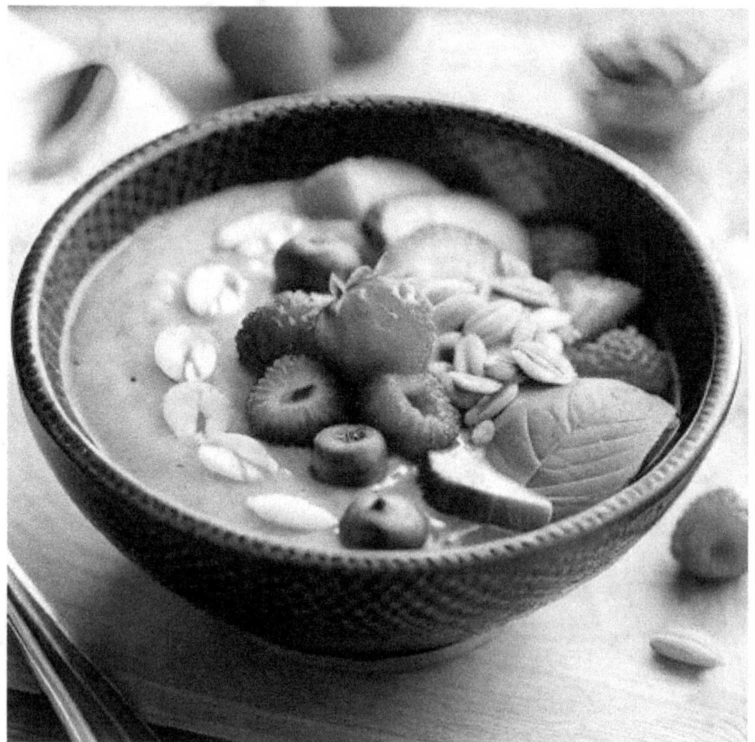

Ingredients:

- 1 cup mixed berries (fresh or frozen)

- 1/2 cup unsweetened almond milk

- 1 handful fresh spinach

- 1 tbsp ground flaxseeds

- 1 small banana, sliced

- 1 tbsp chopped nuts (such as almonds or walnuts)

- 1 tbsp chia seeds

Instructions:

1. Add the mixed berries, almond milk, spinach, and ground flaxseeds to a blender. Blend until smooth.

2. Pour the mixture into a bowl.

3. Top with sliced banana, chopped nuts, and chia seeds.

4. Serve immediately and enjoy!

Avocado Toast with Egg

Ingredients:

- 1 slice whole-grain bread

- 1/2 avocado, mashed

- 1 small tomato, sliced

- 1 egg

- Salt and black pepper to taste

- Fresh herbs (such as cilantro or basil), chopped

Instructions:

1. Toast the whole-grain bread until lightly golden.

2. While the bread is toasting, heat a non-stick skillet over medium heat.

3. Crack the egg into the skillet and cook until the white is set and the yolk is still runny (or cook to your desired doneness).

4. Spread the mashed avocado on top of the toasted bread.

5. Layer the sliced tomato on top of the avocado.

6. Top the tomato with the cooked egg.

7. Sprinkle salt and black pepper to taste.

8. Garnish with fresh herbs.

9. Serve immediately and enjoy!

Oatmeal with Berries

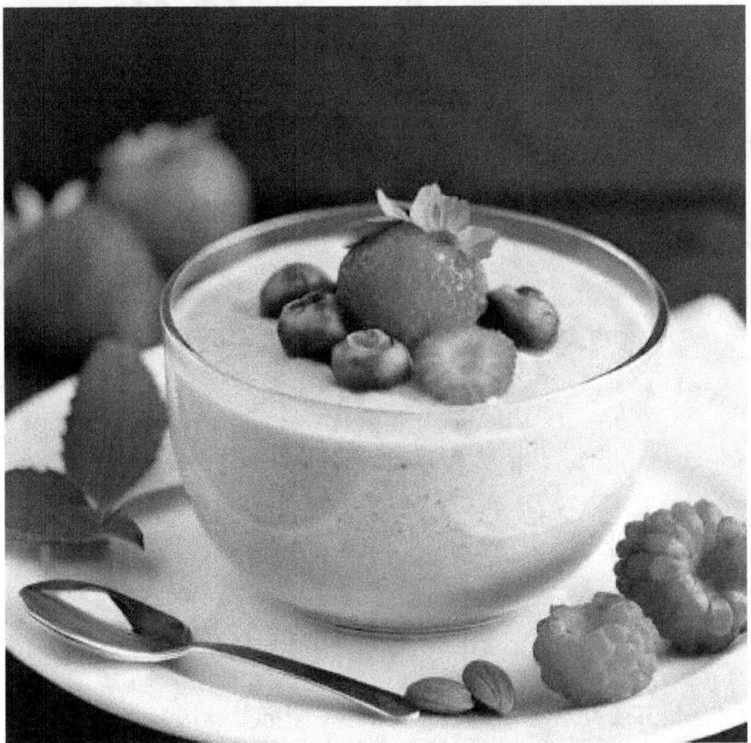

Ingredients:

- 1/2 cup steel-cut oats

- 1 cup unsweetened almond milk

- 1/2 tsp ground cinnamon

- 1/2 cup mixed berries (fresh or frozen)

- 1 tbsp sliced almonds

- 1 tbsp honey

Instructions:

1. In a saucepan, bring the almond milk to a boil.

2. Stir in the steel-cut oats and reduce the heat to a simmer.

3. Cook for 20-25 minutes or until the oats are tender and the liquid is absorbed.

4. Stir in the ground cinnamon.

5. Divide the cooked oatmeal into two bowls.

6. Top with mixed berries, sliced almonds, and a drizzle of honey.

7. Serve warm and enjoy!

Greek Yogurt Parfait

Ingredients:

- 1 cup plain Greek yogurt

- 1 cup mixed fresh fruit (such as strawberries, blueberries, and raspberries)

- 1/2 cup granola

- 2 tbsp peanut butter or almond butter

Instructions:

1. In a tall glass, layer the Greek yogurt, fresh fruit, and granola.

2. Repeat until the glass is full.

3. Top with a dollop of peanut butter or almond butter.

4. Serve immediately and enjoy!

Quinoa Breakfast Bowl

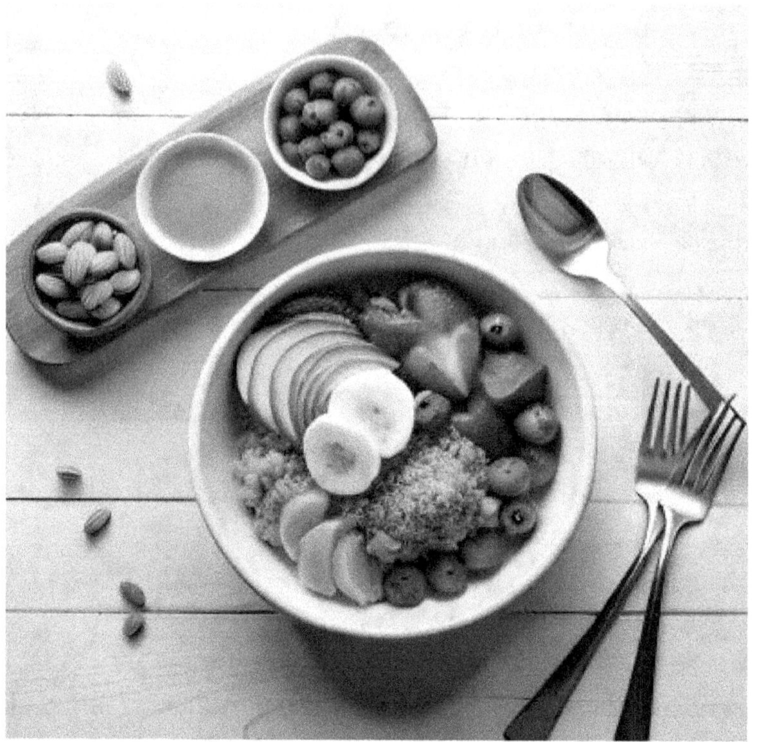

Ingredients:

- 1 cup cooked quinoa

- 1 cup unsweetened almond milk

- 1/2 tsp vanilla extract

- 1 small banana, sliced

- 1 tbsp chopped nuts (such as almonds or walnuts)

* 1 tbsp honey

Instructions:

1. In a saucepan, bring the almond milk to a boil.

2. Stir in the cooked quinoa and vanilla extract.

3. Reduce the heat to a simmer and cook for 5-10 minutes, stirring occasionally, until the liquid is absorbed and the quinoa is heated through.

4. Divide the quinoa mixture into two bowls.

5. Top with sliced banana, chopped nuts, and a drizzle of honey.

6. Serve warm and enjoy!

Veggie Omelet

Ingredients:

* 2 eggs

* 1 tbsp milk
* Salt and black pepper to taste

- 1 tsp olive oil

- 1 cup mixed vegetables (such as spinach, mushrooms, and bell peppers), chopped

Instructions:

1. In a bowl, whisk together the eggs, milk, salt, and black pepper until well combined.

2. Heat the olive oil in a non-stick skillet over medium heat.

3. Add the chopped vegetables and sauté until tender, about 5-7 minutes.

4. Pour the egg mixture over the vegetables.

5. Cook until the eggs are set and the bottom is lightly golden, about 3-4 minutes.

6. Using a spatula, fold the omelet in half.

7. Slide the omelet onto a plate and serve immediately.
8. Enjoy!

Chia Seed Pudding

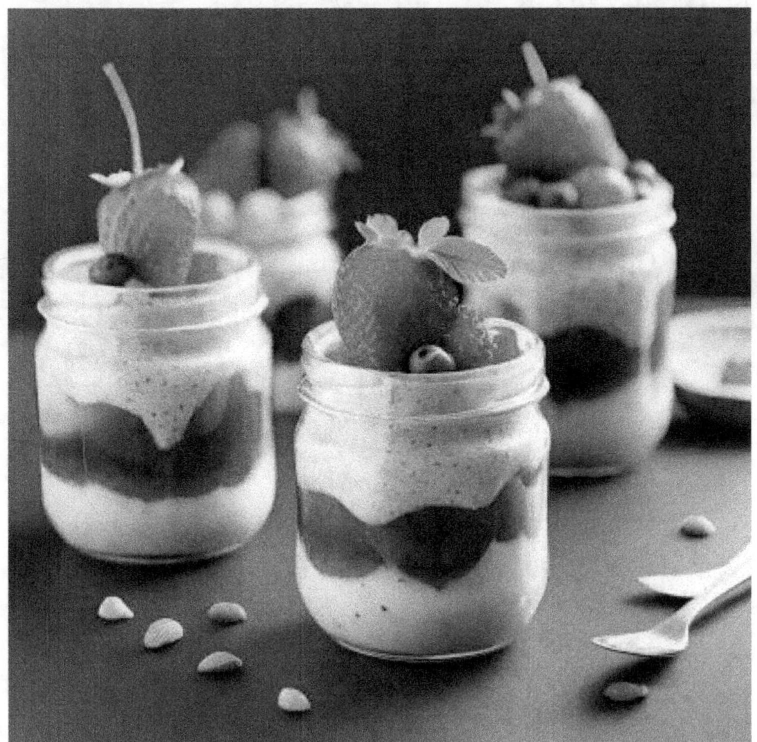

Ingredients:

- 1/4 cup chia seeds

- 1 cup unsweetened almond milk

- 1/2 tsp vanilla extract

- 1 tbsp maple syrup

- Fresh fruit for topping

Instructions:

1. In a bowl, mix together the chia seeds, almond milk, vanilla extract, and maple syrup until well combined.

2. Cover and refrigerate the mixture overnight, or for at least 4 hours, until it thickens into a pudding-like consistency.

3. When ready to serve, divide the chia seed pudding into two bowls.

4. Top with fresh fruit.

5. Serve cold and enjoy!

Breakfast Salad

Ingredients:

- 2 cups mixed greens

- 1/2 cucumber, sliced

- 1/2 cup cherry tomatoes, halved

- 1 avocado, sliced

- 2 eggs, poached

- 1 tbsp olive oil

Instructions:

1. In a large bowl, toss together the mixed greens, sliced cucumber, cherry tomatoes, and avocado.

2. Divide the salad into two plates.

3. Top each salad with a poached egg.

4. Drizzle olive oil over the top.

5. Serve immediately and enjoy!

Sweet Potato Hash

Ingredients:

- 1 large sweet potato, peeled and diced

- 1/2 onion, diced

- 1/2 bell pepper, diced

- 1 garlic clove, minced

- 2 tbsp olive oil

- Salt and black pepper to taste

- 2 eggs, fried

- Chopped herbs for topping (such as parsley or cilantro)

Instructions:

1. In a large skillet, heat the olive oil over medium heat.

2. Add the diced sweet potatoes, onion, bell pepper, and garlic to the skillet.

3. Season with salt and black pepper to taste.

4. Cook, stirring occasionally, until the sweet potatoes are tender and lightly browned, about 15-20 minutes.

5. Divide the sweet potato hash onto two plates.

6. Top each plate with a fried egg.

7. Garnish with chopped herbs.

8. Serve hot and enjoy!

Tofu Scramble

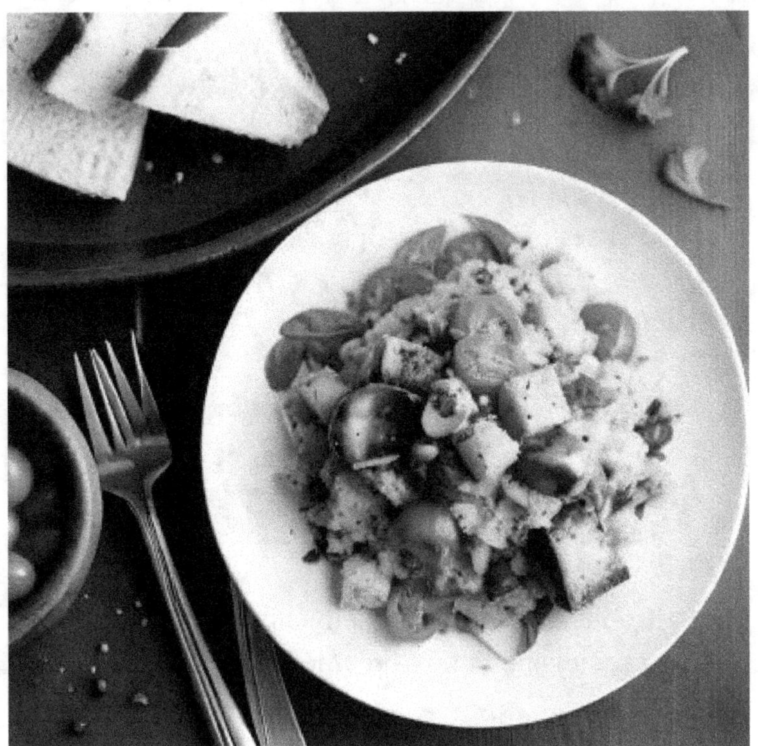

Ingredients:

- 1 block of firm tofu, crumbled

- 1/2 onion, diced

- 1 garlic clove, minced

- 1/2 tsp turmeric

- Salt and black pepper to taste

- 1 cup chopped vegetables (such as spinach, tomatoes, and mushrooms)

- 2 slices of whole-grain bread, toasted

Instructions:

1. In a skillet, heat a little oil over medium heat.

2. Add the crumbled tofu, onion, garlic, turmeric, salt, and black pepper to the skillet.

3. Cook, stirring occasionally, until the tofu is heated through and lightly browned, about 5-7 minutes.

4. Add the chopped vegetables to the skillet and cook until tender, about 3-5 minutes.

5. Divide the tofu scramble onto two plates.

6. Serve with toasted whole-grain bread.

7. Enjoy!

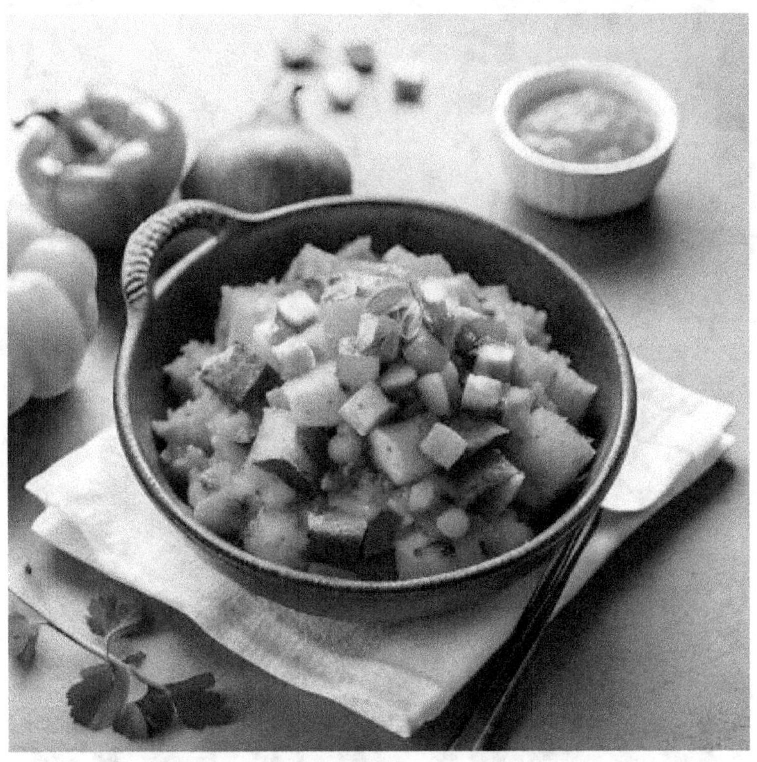

CHAPTER 3

LUNCH RECIPES

Grilled Chicken Salad

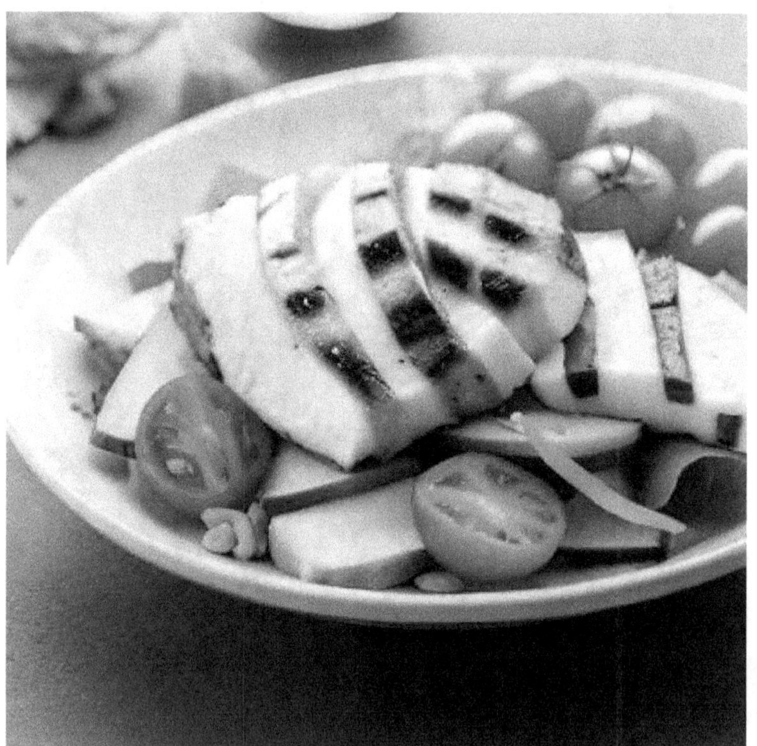

Ingredients:

- 2 boneless, skinless chicken breasts

- Salt and pepper to taste

- 6 cups mixed greens

- 1 cup cherry tomatoes, halved

- 1 cucumber, sliced

- 1/2 cup chopped walnuts

- 1/4 cup balsamic vinaigrette

Instructions

1. Preheat the grill to medium-high heat.

2. Season chicken breasts with salt and pepper.

3. Grill chicken for 5-6 minutes per side or until cooked through.

4. Let chicken cool for a few minutes and then slice into strips.

5. In a large bowl, add mixed greens, cherry tomatoes, cucumber slices, and chopped walnuts.

6. Add chicken strips on top of the salad.

7. Drizzle with balsamic vinaigrette.

8. Toss gently to combine and serve.

Vegetable Soup

Ingredients:

- 2 tablespoons olive oil

- 1 onion, chopped

- 2 cloves garlic, minced

- 2 carrots, chopped

- 2 celery stalks, chopped

- 2 zucchinis, chopped

- 6 cups low-sodium chicken or vegetable broth

- 1 can diced tomatoes

- 1 teaspoon dried thyme

- Salt and pepper to taste

Instructions

1. Heat olive oil in a large pot over medium heat.

2. Add onion, garlic, carrots, celery, and zucchini. Sauté for 5-6 minutes or until vegetables are tender.

3. Add low-sodium chicken or vegetable broth, diced tomatoes, and dried thyme. Bring to a boil.

4. Reduce heat and let simmer for 20-30 minutes or until vegetables are cooked through.

5. Season with salt and pepper to taste.

6. Serve hot and enjoy!

Quinoa and Kale Salad

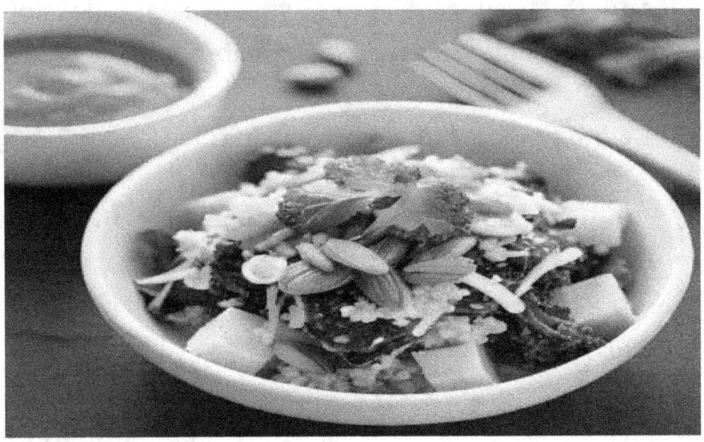

Ingredients:

- 1 cup quinoa

- 2 cups water

- 4 cups kale leaves, torn

- 1/2 cup sliced almonds

- 1 apple, diced

- 1/4 cup honey mustard dressing

Instructions

1. Rinse quinoa in a fine-mesh strainer and drain.

2. In a medium pot, add quinoa and water. Bring to a boil, then reduce heat to low and cover. Cook for 15-20 minutes or until water is absorbed.

3. Let quinoa cool to room temperature.

4. In a large bowl, add kale leaves, sliced almonds, and diced apple.

5. Add cooked quinoa to the bowl.

6. Drizzle with honey mustard dressing and toss to combine.

7. Serve chilled or at room temperature.

Tuna and Avocado Salad

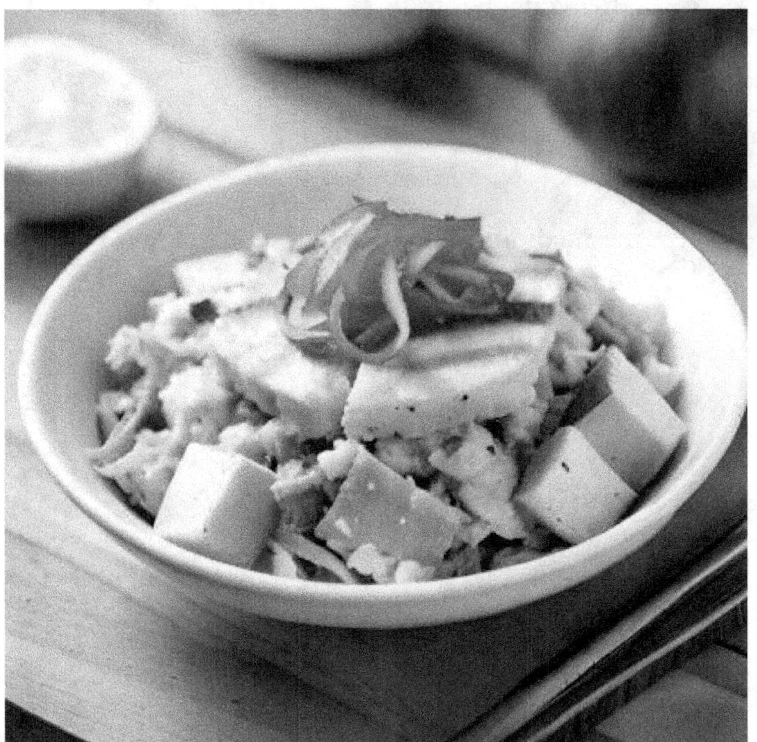

Ingredients:

- 1 can tuna, drained

- 1 avocado, mashed

- 1 celery stalk, chopped

- 1/4 cup diced red onion

- 1 tablespoon lemon juice

- Salt and pepper to taste

- 4 cups mixed greens

Instructions

1. In a medium bowl, add drained tuna and mashed avocado.

2. Add chopped celery, diced red onion, lemon juice, salt, and pepper.

3. Mix well to combine.

4. Serve tuna and avocado salad over a bed of mixed greens.

5. Enjoy!

Greek Yogurt and Berry Parfait

Ingredients:

- 1 cup plain Greek yogurt

- 1 cup mixed berries (such as strawberries, blueberries, and raspberries)

- 1/2 cup granola

- 2 tablespoons honey

Instructions

1. In a glass or bowl, add a layer of Greek yogurt.

2. Add a layer of mixed berries on top of the yogurt.

3. Add a layer of granola on top of the berries.

4. Repeat layering until all ingredients are used.

5. Drizzle honey on top of the parfait.

6. Serve immediately and enjoy!

Lentil Soup

Ingredients:

- 2 tablespoons olive oil

- 1 onion, chopped

- 2 cloves garlic, minced

- 2 carrots, chopped

- 2 cups dry lentils, rinsed

- 6 cups low-sodium chicken or vegetable broth

- 1 can diced tomatoes

- 1 teaspoon dried thyme

- Salt and pepper to taste

Instructions

1. Heat olive oil in a large pot over medium heat.

2. Add onion, garlic, and carrots. Sauté for 5-6 minutes or until vegetables are tender.

3. Add dry lentils, low-sodium chicken or vegetable broth, diced tomatoes, and dried thyme. Bring to a boil.

4. Reduce heat and let simmer for 25-30 minutes or until lentils are cooked through.

5. Season with salt and pepper to taste.

6. Serve hot and enjoy!

Salmon and Sweet Potato Patties

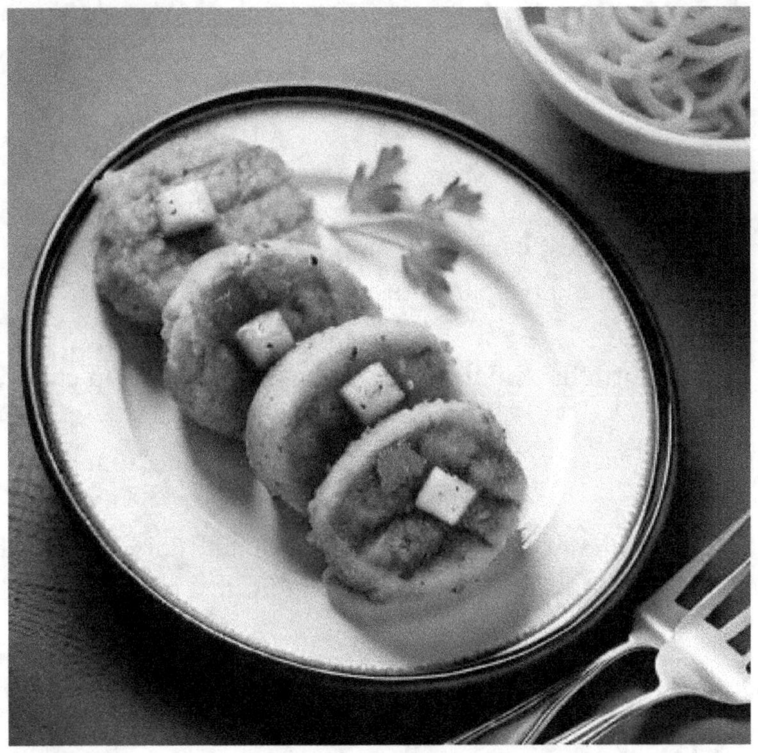

Ingredients:

- 2 medium sweet potatoes, cooked and mashed

- 1 can salmon, drained

- 2 scallions, chopped

- 1 egg

- Salt and pepper to taste

- 2 tablespoons olive oil

Instructions

1. In a large bowl, mix together mashed sweet potatoes, canned salmon, chopped scallions, egg, salt, and pepper until well combined.

2. Form the mixture into patties, about 1/4 cup each.

3. Heat olive oil in a large skillet over medium heat.

4. Add the patties to the skillet and cook for 3-4 minutes on each side or until golden brown.

5. Serve hot and enjoy!

Turkey and Veggie Wrap

Ingredients:

- 1 whole-wheat tortilla

- 2 tablespoons hummus

- 3-4 slices of turkey breast

- 1/4 cup roasted red peppers, sliced

- 1/2 cup sliced cucumber

- 1/2 cup arugula

Instructions

1. Spread hummus on the whole-wheat tortilla.

2. Add sliced turkey breast, roasted red peppers, sliced cucumber, and arugula to the center of the tortilla.

3. Roll up the tortilla and slice into rounds.

4. Serve cold or at room temperature.

5. Enjoy!

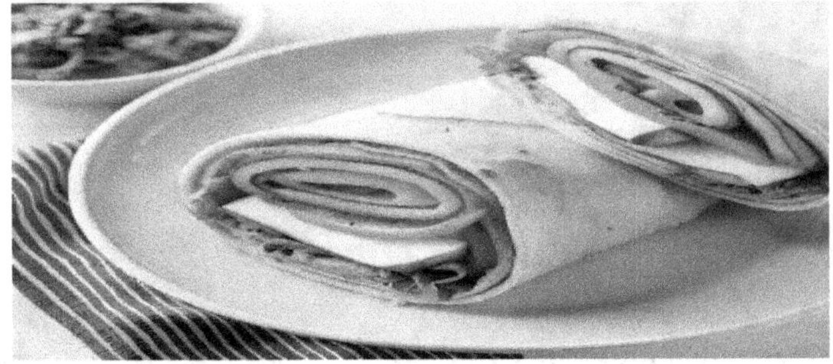

CHAPTER 4

DINNER RECIPES

Baked Salmon

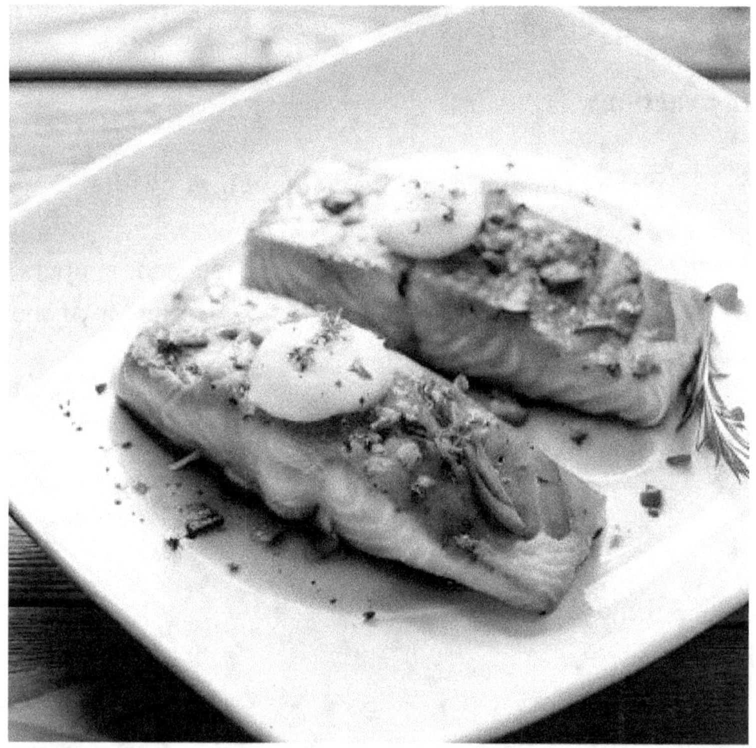

Ingredients:

- 4 salmon filets

- 2 tablespoons olive oil

- 1 tablespoon lemon juice

- 2 garlic cloves, minced

- 2 teaspoons fresh herbs (such as dill or parsley)

- Salt and pepper to taste

Instructions:

1. Preheat the oven to 375°F.

2. Place salmon filets in a baking dish.

3. In a small bowl, whisk together olive oil, lemon juice, garlic, and herbs.

4. Pour the mixture over the salmon filets, making sure they are evenly coated.

5. Season the salmon with salt and pepper to taste.

6. Bake for 12-15 minutes or until the salmon is cooked through.

Roasted Vegetables and Chicken

Ingredients:

- 4 boneless, skinless chicken breasts

- 2 cups chopped vegetables (such as broccoli, cauliflower, carrots, and onions)

- 2 tablespoons olive oil

- 2 teaspoons Italian seasoning

- Salt and pepper to taste

Instructions:

1. Preheat the oven to 400°F.

2. Toss chicken and vegetables with olive oil and seasonings in a large bowl.

3. Spread the mixture on a baking sheet.

4. Roast in the oven for 20-25 minutes or until the vegetables are tender and the chicken is cooked through.

Zucchini Noodles with Tomato Sauce

Ingredients:

- 4 medium zucchini, spiralized

- 2 tablespoons olive oil

- 2 garlic cloves, minced

- 1 (14-ounce) can diced tomatoes

- 1/4 cup chopped onion

- 1 teaspoon Italian seasoning

- Salt and pepper to taste

Instructions:

1. In a large skillet, heat olive oil over medium heat.

2. Add garlic and cook for 1-2 minutes or until fragrant.

3. Add diced tomatoes, onion, Italian seasoning, salt, and pepper to the skillet.

4. Simmer the sauce for 15-20 minutes.

5. Add the zucchini noodles to the skillet and cook for 3-5 minutes or until tender.

6. Serve the zucchini noodles with the tomato sauce
    on top.

Grilled Chicken and Asparagus

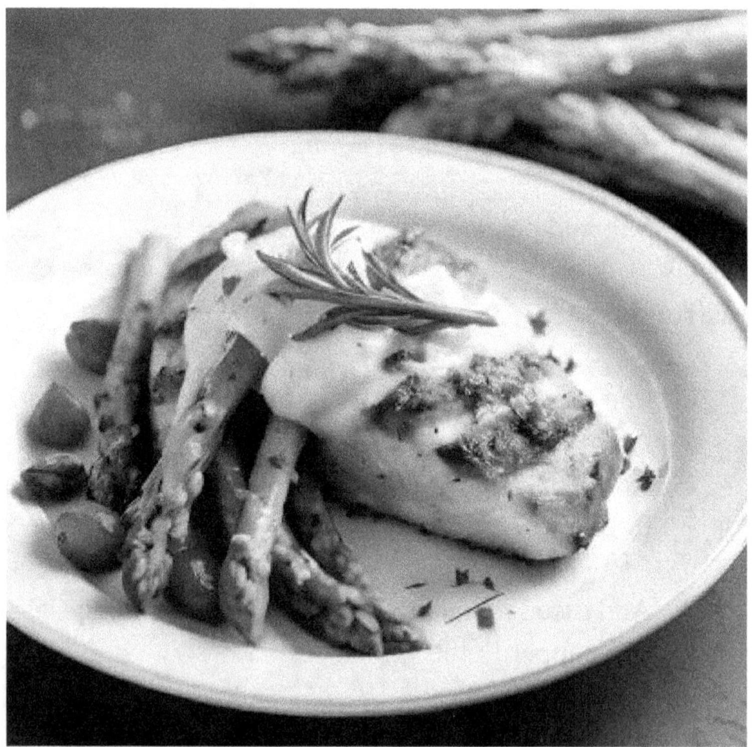

Ingredients:

- 4 boneless, skinless chicken breasts

- 1/4 cup fresh lemon juice

- 3 garlic cloves, minced

- 1 tablespoon chopped fresh herbs (such as rosemary, thyme, or oregano)

- Salt and pepper to taste

- 1 pound asparagus spears, trimmed

- Olive oil for brushing

Instructions:

1. In a large bowl, combine lemon juice, garlic, herbs, salt, and pepper. Add chicken breasts and coat them with the marinade. Cover and refrigerate for at least 30 minutes, or up to 2 hours.

2. Preheat the grill to medium-high heat.

3. Brush the asparagus spears with olive oil and season with salt and pepper. Grill the chicken breasts and asparagus spears until they are cooked through, about 6-8 minutes per side for the chicken and 3-5 minutes for the asparagus.

4. Serve the grilled chicken and asparagus hot with your favorite sides.

Spaghetti Squash with Turkey Bolognese

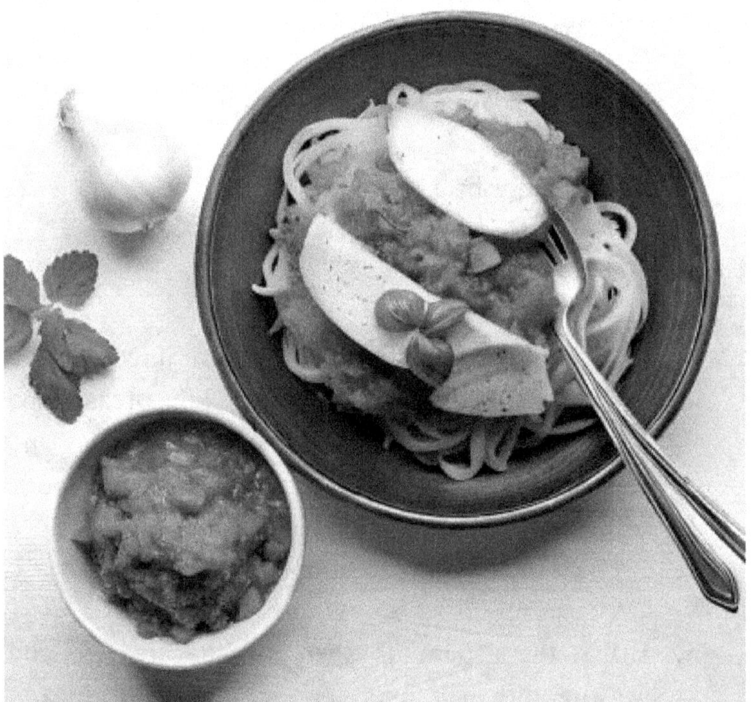

Ingredients:

- 1 medium spaghetti squash, halved and seeded

- 1 pound lean ground turkey

- 1 can (14.5 oz) diced tomatoes, drained

- 1 onion, diced

- 2 garlic cloves, minced

- 1 teaspoon Italian seasoning

- Salt and pepper to taste

- Olive oil for cooking

Instructions:

1. Preheat the oven to 375°F. Line a baking sheet with parchment paper.

2. Brush the cut sides of the spaghetti squash with olive oil and season with salt and pepper. Place the squash halves cut side down on the baking sheet and roast for 45-50 minutes, or until the flesh is tender and easily pierced with a fork.

3. In a large skillet, heat olive oil over medium-high heat. Add the ground turkey and cook until browned, breaking it up with a spoon as it cooks.

4. Add the diced onion and garlic to the skillet and cook until the onion is translucent, about 5 minutes.

5. Add the drained diced tomatoes, Italian seasoning, salt, and pepper to the skillet. Stir to combine and bring to a simmer. Reduce heat and let the sauce simmer for 10-15 minutes, stirring occasionally.

6. Use a fork to scrape the spaghetti squash flesh into a bowl. Divide the spaghetti squash between plates and top with the turkey Bolognese sauce

Quinoa Stuffed Bell Peppers

Ingredients:

- 4 bell peppers, any color

- 1 cup quinoa

- 2 cups water

- 1 tablespoon olive oil

- 1 onion, chopped

- 2 cloves garlic, minced

- 1 cup diced vegetables (such as zucchini, carrots, or mushrooms)

- 1 can (14.5 oz) diced tomatoes, drained

- 1 teaspoon Italian seasoning

- Salt and pepper, to taste

- Optional toppings: shredded cheese, chopped fresh herbs

Instructions:

1. Preheat the oven to 375°F.

2. Cut off the tops of the bell peppers and remove the seeds and membranes. Rinse the peppers and set them aside.

3. In a medium saucepan, bring the quinoa and water to a boil. Reduce the heat to low, cover, and simmer for 15-20 minutes, or until the quinoa is tender and the water is absorbed.

4. While the quinoa cooks, heat the olive oil in a large skillet over medium-high heat. Add the onion and garlic and sauté until the onion is translucent, about 5 minutes.

5. Add the diced vegetables to the skillet and sauté until they are tender, about 5-7 minutes.

6. Stir in the drained diced tomatoes, Italian seasoning, salt, and pepper. Cook for an additional 2-3 minutes.

7. Add the cooked quinoa to the skillet and stir to combine. Remove from heat.

8. Spoon the quinoa mixture into the bell peppers, filling them to the top. Place the peppers upright in a baking dish.

9. Bake for 30-35 minutes, or until the peppers are tender and the filling is hot and bubbly.

10. Optional: top the peppers with shredded cheese and return them to the oven for 5-7 minutes, or until the cheese is melted and bubbly.

11. Serve hot, garnished with chopped fresh herbs if desired. Enjoy!

Eggplant Parmesan

Ingredients:

- 1 large eggplant, sliced into rounds

- 1 cup Italian seasoned breadcrumbs

- 2 eggs, beaten

- 2 cups tomato sauce

- 2 cups shredded mozzarella cheese

- Salt and pepper, to taste

- Olive oil, for baking sheet

Instructions:

1. Preheat the oven to 375°F. Line a large baking sheet with parchment paper and brush with olive oil.

2. Dip each slice of eggplant into the beaten egg, then coat in the breadcrumbs. Place the breaded eggplant slices on the prepared baking sheet.

3. Bake the eggplant slices for 15-20 minutes, or until they are crispy and golden brown.

4. Remove the baking sheet from the oven and spread a thin layer of tomato sauce over each

eggplant slice. Sprinkle shredded mozzarella cheese on top of the sauce.

5. Return the baking sheet to the oven and bake for an additional 10-15 minutes, or until the cheese is melted and bubbly.

6. Serve hot, garnished with fresh basil or parsley if desired.

Lentil and Vegetable Stir Fry

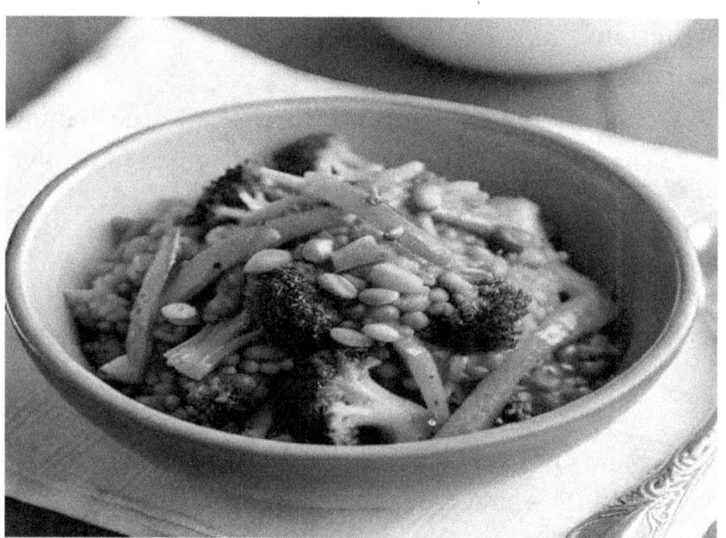

Ingredients:

- 1 cup lentils, cooked

- 1 onion, chopped

- 2 cloves garlic, minced

- 2 bell peppers, sliced

- 2 carrots, sliced

- 1 cup broccoli florets

- 3 tablespoons soy sauce

- 1 teaspoon grated fresh ginger

- 1 tablespoon sesame oil

- Salt and pepper, to taste

- Olive oil, for cooking

Instructions:

1. Heat a large wok or skillet over medium-high heat. Add a drizzle of olive oil and swirl to coat the pan.

2. Add the onion and garlic to the pan and sauté for 2-3 minutes, or until the onion is translucent.

3. Add the sliced bell peppers, carrots, and broccoli to the pan and sauté for 5-7 minutes, or until the vegetables are tender.

4. Add the cooked lentils to the pan and stir to combine.

5. In a small bowl, whisk together the soy sauce, grated ginger, sesame oil, salt, and pepper.

6. Pour the soy sauce mixture over the lentil and vegetable mixture and stir to combine. Cook for an additional 2-3 minutes, or until heated through.

7. Serve hot, garnished with sliced green onions or chopped peanuts if desired.

Turkey Chili

Ingredients:

- 1 lb ground turkey

- 1 onion, chopped

- 3 cloves garlic, minced

- 1 can (14.5 oz) diced tomatoes

- 1 can (15 oz) kidney beans, drained and rinsed

- 2 tablespoons chili powder

- Salt and pepper, to taste

- Olive oil, for cooking

Instructions:

1. Heat a large pot over medium-high heat. Add a drizzle of olive oil and swirl to coat the pot.

2. Add the ground turkey to the pot and brown for 5-7 minutes, breaking up any large pieces with a wooden spoon.

3. Add the chopped onion and minced garlic to the pot and sauté for 2-3 minutes, or until the onion is translucent.

4. Add the diced tomatoes, kidney beans, chili powder, salt, and pepper to the pot. Stir to combine.

5. Bring the chili to a simmer and cook for 30-40 minutes, stirring occasionally.

6. Serve hot, garnished with shredded cheese and chopped fresh cilantro if desired.

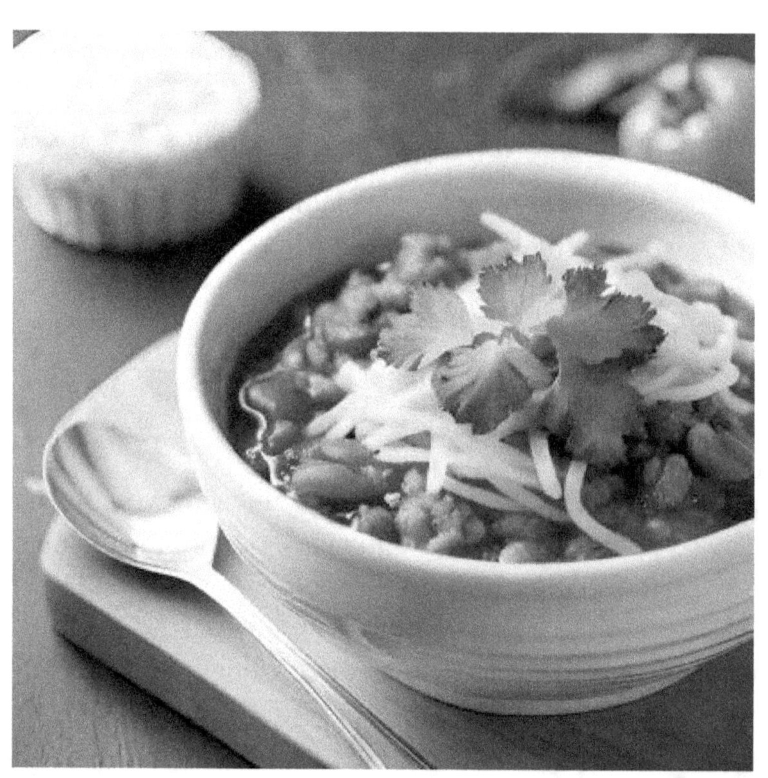

CHAPTER 5

SNACK AND DESSERT RECIPES

Baked Cinnamon Apple Chips

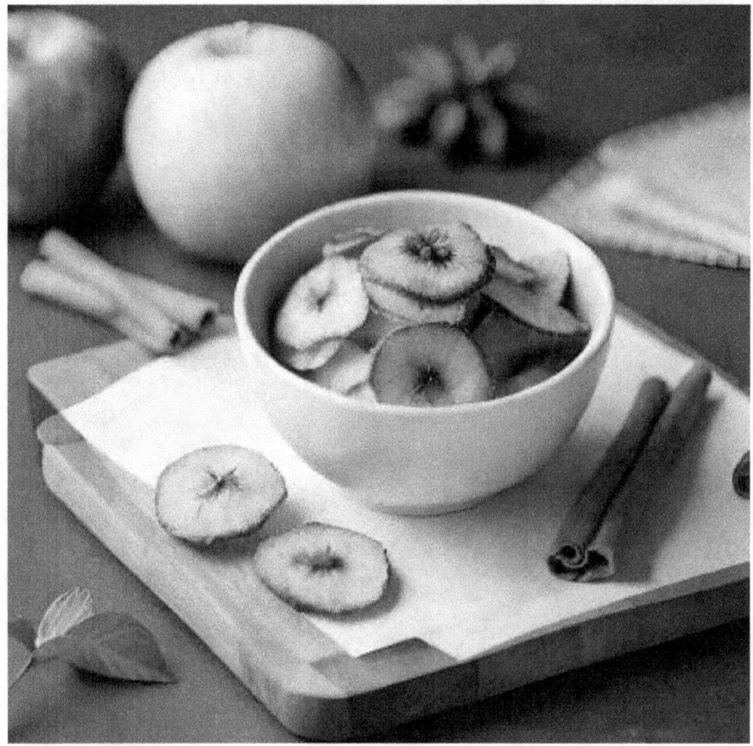

Ingredients:

- 2 medium-sized apples

- 1 tablespoon cinnamon

Instructions:

1. Preheat the oven to 200°F.

2. Thinly slice the apples using a mandolin or sharp knife.

3. Arrange the apple slices on a baking sheet lined with parchment paper.

4. Sprinkle cinnamon over the apple slices.

5. Bake in the oven for 2-3 hours or until crispy.

6. Allow to cool and serve.

Chocolate Avocado Pudding

Ingredients:

- 2 ripe avocados

- 1/2 cup unsweetened cocoa powder

- 1/2 cup pure maple syrup

- 1 teaspoon vanilla extract

- 1/4 teaspoon sea salt

Instructions:

1. Cut the avocados in half, remove the pit, and scoop the flesh into a food processor or blender.

2. Add cocoa powder, maple syrup, vanilla extract, and sea salt to the food processor or blender.

3. Blend until the mixture is smooth and creamy.

4. Transfer the pudding into small bowls and chill in the refrigerator for at least 30 minutes before serving.

Quinoa and Vegetable Salad

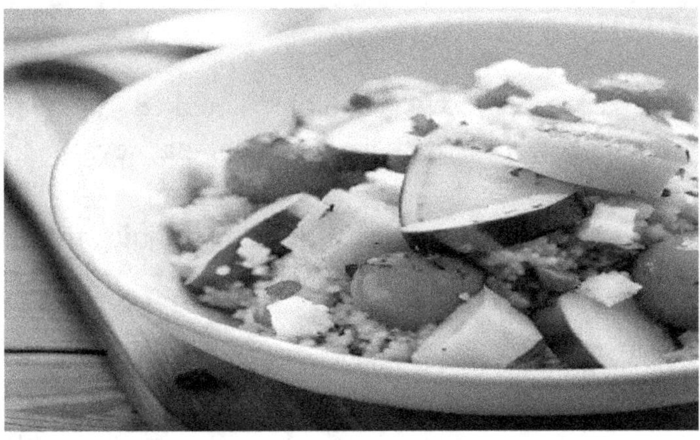

Ingredients:

- 1 cup cooked quinoa

- 1/2 cup diced cucumber

- 1/2 cup diced tomato

- 1/2 cup diced bell pepper

- 1/4 cup chopped fresh parsley

- 1/4 cup crumbled feta cheese

- 2 tablespoons olive oil

- 2 tablespoons lemon juice

- Salt and pepper to taste

Instructions:

1. In a large bowl, combine cooked quinoa, cucumber, tomato, bell pepper, and parsley.

2. Add feta cheese, olive oil, and lemon juice to the bowl.

3. Toss until all ingredients are well combined.

4. Season with salt and pepper to taste.

5. Serve chilled.

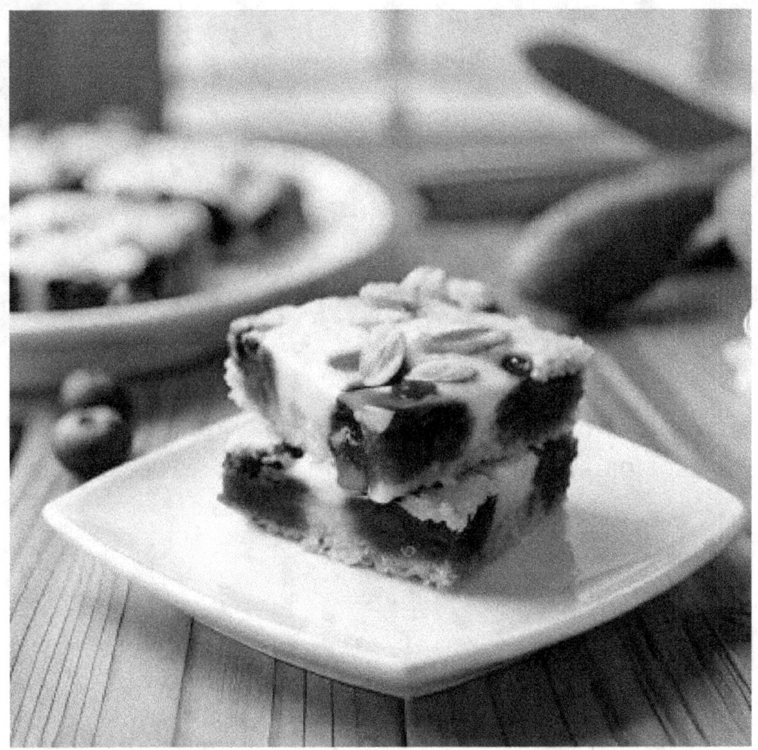

Ingredients:

- 2 cups rolled oats

- 1/2 cup almond flour

- 1/4 cup coconut oil

- 1/4 cup pure maple syrup

- 1/4 teaspoon sea salt

- 1 cup fresh blueberries

Instructions:

1. Preheat the oven to 350°F.

2. Line an 8x8 inch baking dish with parchment paper.

3. In a large mixing bowl, combine rolled oats, almond flour, coconut oil, maple syrup, and sea salt.

4. Stir until well combined.

5. Fold in the fresh blueberries.

6. Transfer the mixture to the prepared baking dish.

7. Bake in the oven for 20-25 minutes or until golden brown.

8. Allow to cool and cut into bars.

Sweet Potato Brownies

Ingredients:

- 1 large sweet potato, cooked and mashed
- 1/2 cup almond flour
- 1/2 cup unsweetened cocoa powder
- 1/2 cup pure maple syrup
- 1/4 cup coconut oil
- 2 eggs
- 1 teaspoon vanilla extract
- 1/4 teaspoon sea salt

Instructions:

1. Preheat the oven to 350°F.

2. Grease an 8x8 inch baking dish with coconut oil.

3. In a large mixing bowl, combine mashed sweet potato, almond flour, cocoa powder, maple syrup, coconut oil, eggs, vanilla extract, and sea salt.

4. Stir until well combined.

5. Transfer the mixture to the prepared baking dish.

6. Bake in the oven for 25-30 minutes or until a
    toothpick comes out clean when inserted in

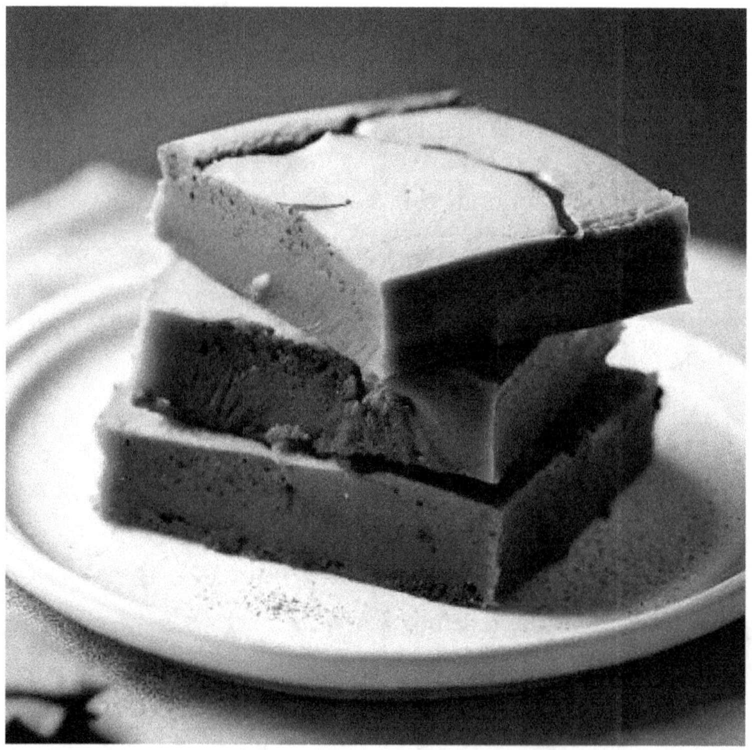

CHAPTER 6

21 DAYS MEAL PLAN

Day 1:

Breakfast: Oatmeal with mixed berries and almond milk
Snack: Apple slices with almond butter
Lunch: Quinoa and lentil salad with mixed greens and avocado
Snack: Carrots with hummus
Dinner: Grilled salmon with roasted vegetables and brown rice

Day 2:

Breakfast: Greek yogurt with sliced banana and walnuts
Snack: Trail mix with dried fruit and nuts
Lunch: Chickpea and vegetable stir-fry with brown rice
Snack: Edamame
Dinner: Chicken and vegetable curry with quinoa

Day 3:

Breakfast: Smoothie with spinach, frozen berries, and almond milk
Snack: Pear slices with cashew butter
Lunch: Turkey and vegetable wrap with mixed greens

Snack: Roasted pumpkin seeds
Dinner: Baked sweet potato with black beans, salsa, and avocado

Day 4:

Breakfast: Scrambled eggs with spinach and whole grain toast
Snack: Orange slices with almonds
Lunch: Lentil soup with mixed greens
Snack: Yogurt with mixed berries
Dinner: Grilled chicken with roasted vegetables and brown rice

Day 5:

Breakfast: Overnight oats with chia seeds and mixed berries
Snack: Trail mix with dried fruit and nuts
Lunch: Tuna salad with mixed greens and whole grain crackers
Snack: Hummus with cucumber slices
Dinner: Beef and vegetable stir-fry with brown rice

Day 6:

Breakfast: Whole grain toast with avocado and sliced tomato

Snack: Apple slices with almond butter
Lunch: Vegetable and quinoa soup with mixed greens
Snack: Mixed nuts
Dinner: Baked salmon with roasted vegetables and sweet potato

Day 7:

Breakfast: Smoothie with spinach, frozen berries, and almond milk
Snack: Carrots with hummus
Lunch: Grilled chicken and vegetable wrap with mixed greens
Snack: Roasted pumpkin seeds
Dinner: Quinoa and vegetable stir-fry with tofu

Day 8:

Breakfast: Greek yogurt with sliced banana and walnuts
Snack: Trail mix with dried fruit and nuts
Lunch: Lentil and vegetable salad with mixed greens
Snack: Edamame
Dinner: Baked chicken with roasted vegetables and brown rice

Day 9:

Breakfast: Oatmeal with mixed berries and almond milk

Snack: Pear slices with cashew butter
Lunch: Tuna and vegetable wrap with mixed greens
Snack: Mixed nuts
Dinner: Beef and vegetable curry with quinoa

Day 10:

Breakfast: Scrambled eggs with spinach and whole grain toast
Snack: Orange slices with almonds
Lunch: Chickpea and vegetable soup with mixed greens
Snack: Yogurt with mixed berries
Dinner: Grilled salmon with roasted vegetables and brown rice

Day 11:

Breakfast: Smoothie with spinach, frozen berries, and almond milk
Snack: Apple slices with almond butter
Lunch: Chicken and vegetable wrap with mixed greens
Snack: Roasted pumpkin seeds
Dinner: Quinoa and vegetable stir-fry with tofu

Day 12:

Breakfast: Greek yogurt with sliced banana and walnuts
Snack: Trail mix with dried fruit and nuts

Lunch: Lentil and vegetable salad with mixed greens
Snack: Edamame
Dinner: Baked chicken with roasted vegetables and brown rice

Day 13:

Breakfast: Overnight oats with chia seeds and mixed berries
Snack: Carrots with hummus
Lunch: Quinoa and lentil salad with mixed greens and avocado
Snack: Mixed nuts
Dinner: Grilled chicken with roasted vegetables and brown rice

Day 14:

Breakfast: Smoothie with spinach, frozen berries, and almond milk
Snack: Apple slices with almond butter
Lunch: Vegetable and quinoa soup with mixed greens
Snack: Roasted pumpkin seeds
Dinner: Baked salmon with roasted vegetables and sweet potato

Day 15:

Breakfast: Scrambled eggs with spinach and whole grain toast
Snack: Pear slices with cashew butter
Lunch: Turkey and vegetable wrap with mixed greens
Snack: Yogurt with mixed berries
Dinner: Beef and vegetable stir-fry with brown rice

Day 16:

Breakfast: Oatmeal with mixed berries and almond milk
Snack: Trail mix with dried fruit and nuts
Lunch: Chickpea and vegetable stir-fry with brown rice
Snack: Edamame
Dinner: Grilled salmon with roasted vegetables and brown rice

Day 17:

Breakfast: Greek yogurt with sliced banana and walnuts
Snack: Carrots with hummus
Lunch: Lentil and vegetable salad with mixed greens
Snack: Mixed nuts
Dinner: Quinoa and vegetable stir-fry with tofu

Day 18:

Breakfast: Smoothie with spinach, frozen berries, and almond milk

Snack: Apple slices with almond butter
Lunch: Chicken and vegetable wrap with mixed greens
Snack: Roasted pumpkin seeds
Dinner: Baked sweet potato with black beans, salsa, and avocado

Day 19:

Breakfast: Overnight oats with chia seeds and mixed berries
Snack: Pear slices with cashew butter
Lunch: Vegetable and lentil soup with mixed greens
Snack: Yogurt with mixed berries
Dinner: Beef and vegetable curry with quinoa

Day 20:

Breakfast: Scrambled eggs with spinach and whole grain toast
Snack: Orange slices with almonds
Lunch: Tuna and vegetable wrap with mixed greens
Snack: Hummus with cucumber slices
Dinner: Grilled chicken with roasted vegetables and brown rice

Day 21:

Breakfast: Oatmeal with mixed berries and almond milk

Snack: Trail mix with dried fruit and nuts
Lunch: Quinoa and vegetable salad with mixed greens and avocado
Snack: Mixed nuts
Dinner: Baked salmon with roasted vegetables and brown rice

Grocery shopping and meal prep can be challenging for breast cancer patients during treatment, but with some planning and preparation, it can be made easier. Here are some grocery shopping and meal prep tips for breast cancer patients:

1. Make a grocery list: Before heading to the grocery store, patients should make a list of the foods they need for their meals and snacks. This can help them stay on track and avoid impulse purchases.

2. Shop the perimeter of the store: The perimeter of the grocery store typically contains fresh produce, meat, and dairy products, which are generally healthier options. Patients can focus on these areas of the store and avoid processed foods and snacks.

3. Consider online grocery shopping: Online grocery shopping can be a convenient option for patients

who may have limited mobility or energy during treatment. Many grocery stores offer online ordering and delivery options.

4. Prep ingredients in advance: Patients can save time and energy by prepping ingredients in advance, such as chopping vegetables, cooking grains, or marinating meat. This can make meal preparation quicker and easier.

5. Use convenience foods: While fresh, whole foods are generally the healthiest option, patients can also make use of convenience foods such as pre-cut vegetables, canned beans, or pre-cooked chicken to make meal preparation easier.

6. Cook in bulk: Patients can save time and energy by cooking meals in bulk and freezing them for later use. This can be especially helpful for days when patients may not have the energy to cook.

7. Make use of slow cookers and instant pots: Slow cookers and instant pots can be great tools for meal preparation, as they allow patients to prepare meals with minimal effort. Patients can find many healthy slow cooker and instant pot recipes online.

By incorporating these grocery shopping and meal prep tips, breast cancer patients can make meal preparation easier and more manageable during treatment.

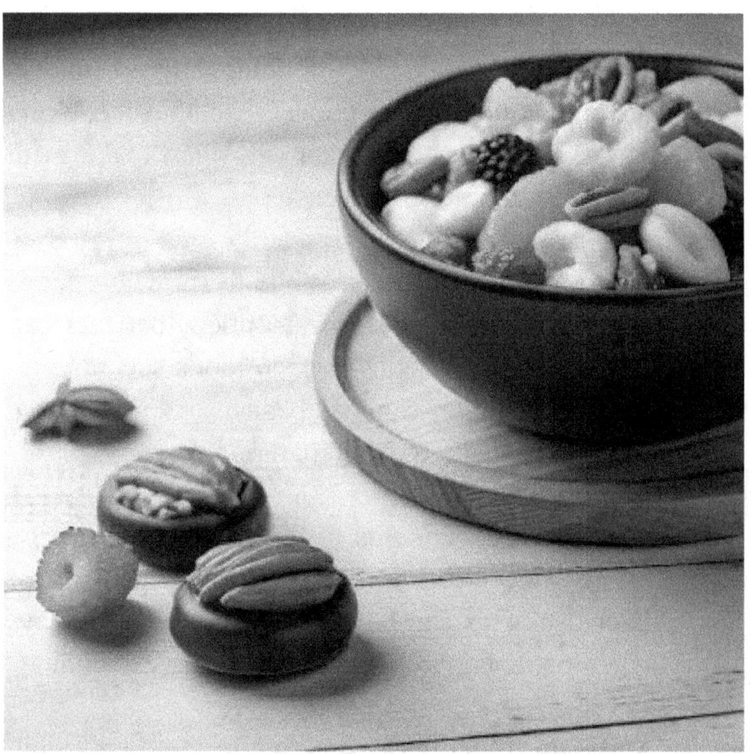

CONCLUSION

In conclusion, a healthy diet can be very helpful for maintaining the health and wellbeing of breast cancer patients while they are receiving treatment. Patients can improve their general health and control treatment side effects by concentrating on nutrient-dense diets, restricting or avoiding particular foods, and implementing good meal planning practices. To develop a customized meal plan that suits their unique requirements and preferences, patients should consult with their doctor or a qualified dietitian. Breast cancer sufferers can improve their overall quality of life and strengthen their body's ability to fight the disease by making nutrition a priority while undergoing cancer treatment.

Additional resources and cookbooks

If you're looking for more resources and cookbooks related to the breast cancer diet, here are some options to consider:

1. "The Breast Cancer Survival Cookbook: Delicious, Nutritious Recipes for During and After Treatment" by Dr. John A. West, PhD and Chef Rebecca Katz
This cookbook provides over 100 recipes specifically designed to support breast cancer

patients during and after treatment. It also includes nutritional guidance and advice from a breast cancer surgeon and an expert chef.

2. "The Cancer-Fighting Kitchen: Nourishing, Big-Flavor Recipes for Cancer Treatment and Recovery" by Rebecca Katz and Mat EdelsonWhile not specific to breast cancer, this cookbook provides a wealth of information and recipes designed to support cancer patients and survivors through nutrition. It includes advice on meal planning, grocery shopping, and preparing nourishing meals.

3. The American Cancer Society: provides a wide range of resources related to nutrition and cancer, including guidelines for healthy eating during and after treatment, recipes, and advice on managing side effects.

4. The National Cancer Institute: provides resources related to nutrition and cancer, including information on key nutrients, meal planning, and tips for grocery shopping and meal prep.